ISOMETRIC CORE EXERCISES FOR SENIORS

A Comprehensive Guide to Isometric Core Exercises for seniors to Enhance Stability, Mobility, and Overall Well-being.

VIVIAN JERNIGAN

Vivian Jernigan

Vivian Jernigan

TABLE OF CONTENTS

Vivian Jernigan

INTRODUCTION

Hi there! Here's ***"Isometric Core Exercises for seniors"*** your one-stop resource for strengthening your core and feeling your best. Let's explore the importance of core stability, the amazing advantages of isometric workouts, and how this book will become your new best friend at the gym.

Now imagine that you are getting out of bed in the morning or that you are reaching up to retrieve something from a high shelf. What makes it easier for you to carry out those routine tasks? Your central muscles! These are the muscles that surround your core and help you remain balanced, steady, and limber. However, as we age, these muscles may begin to weaken, which can result in aches, pains, and even falls. But do not worry! This book is meant to support you in maintaining the strength and readiness of your core muscles.

The Amazing Advantages of Isometric Training

Let's now discuss isometric workouts, also known as the "superhero moves" of the fitness industry. Although these exercises may seem sophisticated, they're actually very easy to perform and very beneficial, particularly for seniors. Isometric exercises include keeping a position without moving, in contrast to other workouts that require a lot of leaping or lifting large weights. For those of us who wish to maintain an active lifestyle without running the danger of injury, this translates to reduced tension on your muscles and joints.

The truly amazing thing is that isometric workouts are incredibly beneficial to your body. They strengthen your core muscles while also enhancing your stability, balance, and posture. They're also quite adaptable! These may be done anywhere, whether it's at home, in the park, or even in front of the TV. Everywhere you go, it's like having your own little gym!

How to Use this Book

Now, let's discuss what to anticipate from **"Isometric Core Exercises for seniors."** We'll start by breaking down all the information you require to get started safely. We have you covered for everything from correctly warming up to paying attention to your body's cues. Next, we'll delve deeper into your core muscles, explaining what they are, why they matter, and how to maintain optimal health.

It's time to move on after that! We'll guide you through a range of isometric core workouts, including lower back strengthening and abs and obliques targeting routines. If you're new to exercising, don't worry; we'll provide you with lots of advice and adjustments based on your level of fitness. We'll even include some sample routines and workouts to help you stay motivated.

Did I also mention that we'll talk about maintaining motivation, remaining healthy, and resolving typical problems? Indeed, this book serves as your one-stop resource for everything related to core strength and fitness.

Now, find a comfortable place to relax, get a glass of water if you want, and let's begin our journey to a more confident, colorful version of ourselves. This is something you can handle!

Chapter 1

Understanding Isometric Exercises

Greetings from Chapter 1! Let's explore the amazing world of isometric workouts and see how seniors like you may increase general well-being, strengthen their bodies, and improve their stability with these exercises. You will have a firm understanding of isometric exercises, their advantages for senior citizens, and safe and efficient methods for performing them by the end of this chapter.

What are Isometric Exercises

Strength training exercises known as isometrics require you to maintain a static posture without moving your joints. Isometric workouts, as opposed to dynamic exercises, concentrate on activating particular muscle groups through resistance-based contractions. Imagine pushing against a brick wall; even though you are applying force, the wall remains stationary. Isometric exercises are frequently performed with planks, wall sits, and static lunges.

The adaptability of isometric exercises is one of their best features. They require little to no equipment, and they can be done almost anyplace. For seniors who might not have access to a gym or who would rather work out in the comfort of their own home, this makes them a great choice. Isometric exercises are very easy on the joints due to their moderate impact, which lowers the chance of damage.

Benefits for Seniors

For elders, isometric workouts have many advantages. Above all, they're a great way to increase muscle strength and endurance, which is essential for preserving independence and carrying out daily tasks with easily. Isometric exercises help older persons feel more stable and balanced by using their core muscles, which lowers their risk of falls and injuries.

Targeting particular muscle groups without overstretching the joints is another benefit of isometric exercises. They are therefore perfect for elderly people who may have arthritis or other joint problems. Furthermore, you can simply add isometric workouts into your daily routine whether you're at home, at the park, or on vacation because they don't require any particular equipment.

Safety Considerations

Safety should always come first when exercising, especially for elderly people. See your doctor before beginning an isometric exercise regimen, particularly if you have any underlying medical ailments or concerns. If isometric exercises seem like a good fit for you, your doctor can advise you on how to begin safely.

Exercises that are isometric require you to pay attention to your body and not push yourself too hard. In the event that you feel any pain or discomfort, cease right away and get medical advice. To lower the chance of injury and prepare your muscles and joints for movement, it's also crucial to warm up before exercising. Usually, a five to ten minute warm-up that involves light stretching or walking is adequate.

When performing isometric exercises, it's important to focus on good form and technique in addition to warming up. In addition to lowering the chance of strain or damage, this will assist the workouts work as hard as possible.

If you're not sure how to carry out a specific activity, think considering consulting a licensed physical therapist or fitness teacher who can offer direction and encouragement.

You may reap the advantages of isometric workouts while lowering your risk of injury by paying attention to these safety precautions and approaching them mindfully and cautiously. Always remember that it's best to begin slowly and build up to a more intense workout as your strength and confidence rise.

Chapter 2

Getting Started Safely

Greetings from Chapter 2! We'll look at how to safely and successfully get started on the path to stronger core muscles in this chapter. Everything from getting ready for exercise to warming up correctly and paying attention to your body's cues will be covered. You'll feel secure and prepared to start your isometric exercise regimen by the end of this chapter.

Getting Ready for Exercise

It's crucial to give oneself enough time to emotionally and physically prepare before beginning any new fitness regimen. Begin by establishing reasonable objectives for yourself. What do you want to accomplish with your isometric exercises? Having specific goals can help you stay motivated and focused, whether your goal is to feel more energised, increase your core strength, or improve your balance.

Next, evaluate your degree of fitness at the moment and any potential limits. Are there any injuries or health issues you should be aware of? If so, discuss the best course of action with your physician or a certified fitness specialist. In order to prevent overexertion or damage, always pay attention to your body's signals and work within your limits.

Techniques for Warm-Up and Cool-Down

It's time to warm up those muscles and joints so they're ready for activity when you're ready to move. An appropriate warm-up promotes flexibility, lowers the chance of injury, and increases blood flow to your muscles. To get your heart rate up and your muscles warm, start with five to ten minutes of light cardiovascular exercise, such walking or cycling.

Remember to cool down and stretch your muscles after your workout to help avoid soreness and stiffness. Stretching should be concentrated on, with each stretch being held for

15 to 30 seconds without bouncing, the muscles you worked during your workout. Adding a stretching and cool-down to your workouts will assist increase range of motion and flexibility, which will make it simpler to move and do daily tasks.

Listening to your Body: Signs to watch for

It's crucial to pay attention to your body's cues and make necessary adjustments during your workout. As soon as you feel any pain, lightheadedness, or discomfort, stop working out and take a break. These can indicate exhaustion or a medical condition that needs to be checked out.

In a similar vein, don't be afraid to take a day off or reduce the intensity of your workout if you're feeling worn out. It's crucial to find a balance between pushing yourself and knowing when to back off since pushing yourself too hard might result in burnout and injury.

You may exercise safely and efficiently, ensuring long-term success and happiness in your fitness journey, by learning to listen to and honor your body's requirements.

Chapter 3

Core Muscles and their Functions

We'll examine the core muscles and their vital roles in the body in more detail in this chapter. Gaining an understanding of the structure of your core will enable you to target these muscles during isometric workouts, improving your strength and stability.

Anatomy of the Core

Your entire body's stability and support come from the intricate network of muscles that make up your core, which is much more than just your abs. The rectus abdominis (the front of the abdomen), obliques (the sides of the abdomen), transverse abdominis (the deep abdominal muscles), and erector spinae (the muscles along the spine) are some of the groups into which these muscles are split.

Your spine, pelvis, and torso are supported by each of these muscle groups in a different way, which enables you to move effectively and safely in all directions. You may improve your overall stability and posture by strengthening your core from all sides by focusing on each of these muscle groups with targeted exercises.

The Functions of the Core Muscles in Everyday Activities

Almost every movement you perform throughout the day, including bending, lifting, twisting, and turning, uses your core muscles. They aid in the transfer of force between your upper and lower bodies and serve as the basis for all other motions. Simple activities like getting out of bed, collecting groceries, or playing with your grandchildren can become difficult or even painful if you don't have a strong core.

A strong core is necessary to support everyday tasks as well as to maintain good posture and alignment, which lowers the risk of back pain and injuries. Your general quality of life will increase as a result of strengthening your core muscles, which will also make you feel more balanced and solid.

You'll be more prepared to target your core muscles throughout your isometric exercise program now that you have a greater grasp of them and how they work. We'll go into particular isometric exercises in the upcoming chapter that will help you develop a stronger, more resilient core by strengthening each of these muscle groups.

Vivian Jernigan

Chapter 4

Essential Equipment and Space

We'll look at the space requirements and necessary equipment for isometric core exercises in this chapter. The proper equipment may make all the difference in your workout, whether you're working out at home, the gym, or on the go. Let's get started and prepare you for success!

Minimal Equipment Needed

Isometric workouts have the advantage of requiring little equipment, which means that almost everyone can perform them. In fact, with just your body weight and a few basic props, you can execute a lot of isometric exercises. Common pieces of equipment for isometric workouts include:

- **Exercise mat:** Offers support and padding for exercises performed on the floor.
- Exercises with a stability ball become more unstable, which increases the difficulty for your core muscles.
- **Resistance bands:** Increase the resistance in exercises to make them more difficult and efficient.
- **Wall or stable surface:** Offers assistance for workouts like plank variations and wall sits.

These are only a handful of the tools you can utilize to improve your isometric training. It's crucial to locate equipment that suits your needs and preferences, so feel free to get creative and use whatever props you have on hand.

Organizing Your Home Workout Area

Establishing a special area at home for exercising will support your motivation and attention to reach your fitness objectives. Locate a peaceful, clutter-free space with enough space for you to walk around comfortably before you do anything else. Your workout area should ideally have adequate lighting, ventilation, and room to stretch out a mat or complete exercises without running into walls or furniture.

After you've located the ideal location, think about incorporating some inspirational features to keep you motivated while working out. Anything from motivational sayings or images to lively music or your go-to exercise equipment could be this. You may increase the fun and satisfaction of your workouts by personalizing your training area.

Mobile Exercises

You can get in a brief isometric workout anywhere, even if you're on the go or don't have access to a regular gym facility. Isometric exercises are ideal for on-the-go workouts since they can be done with just your body weight and a little space.

You can easily get in a quick workout to keep your energy levels high and your core muscles active, whether you're waiting for a flight at the airport, in a hotel room, or at the park. Additionally, adding frequent activity to your daily schedule will help counteract the detrimental effects of extended sitting and enhance your general health and wellbeing.

You may use isometric core exercises to help you reach your fitness objectives if you set up a dedicated exercise area at home and learn how to modify your routines to match your schedule.

Chapter 5

Isometric Core Exercises

We'll explore a range of isometric core exercises in this chapter that are intended to work your lower back, oblique, and abdominal muscles. Your core will become stronger, more stable, and more resilient with the aid of these workouts, which will also help you maintain better posture and lower your chance of injury. Now let's get going!

Exercises for Strengthening the Abdomen

- **Plank:** Take a push-up stance, placing your hands squarely beneath your shoulders and aligning your torso so that your head and heels make a straight line. As long as you can, maintain this posture while using your core muscles to prevent your hips from heaving or sagging.

- **Leg Lift Hold:** Assume a prone position and raise your legs straight up toward the ceiling. Lower your legs toward the floor until you feel your lower back beginning to arch, then place your hands under your lower back for support. As long as you can, maintain this posture with your core active.

Exercises for Oblique

Strengthening

- **Side Plank:** Assume a side laying position with your legs stacked on top of one another and your elbow directly beneath your shoulder. Raise your hips off the floor so that your head and heels are in a straight line. As long as you can, maintain this posture; then, switch sides.
- **Russian Twist Hold:** Assume a seated position with your feet flat on the floor and your knees bent. Using your sit bones for balance, slant your back a little and raise your feet off the ground. Engage

your oblique muscles by twisting your body from side to side while holding a weight or medicine ball in front of your chest.

Exercises to Strengthen Your Lower Back

- **Superman Hold:** Extend your arms high and your legs straight behind you while lying face down on the ground. Squeeze your glutes and lower back muscles to rise as high as you can while raising your arms, chest, and legs off the ground. After a little period of holding this position, descend once more.
- Start on your hands and knees, placing your wrists just beneath your shoulders and your knees beneath your hips, to do the bird dog hold. Make a straight line from your fingertips to your toes by extending your right arm forward and your left leg back. After a few seconds, hold this posture and swap sides.

These are just a few training routines that you can use that include isometric core workouts. When performing any exercise, keep in mind that keeping good form and using your core muscles will optimize its effectiveness and reduce the risk of injury.

Chapter 6

Full Body Integration

Greetings from Chapter 6! We'll look at how to include isometric core exercises in full-body workouts to enhance functional strength, stability, and balance in this chapter. You'll improve your general health and well-being in addition to strengthening your core by adding these workouts into your program. Now let's get started!

Exercises to Boost Stability and Balance

- **Single-Leg Balance:** Place your hands on your hips and stand on one leg with your knee slightly bent. To keep your balance, contract your core muscles, and try to stay in this posture for as long as you can. Repeat after switching legs.

- **Bosu Ball Squat Hold:** Place your arms out in front of you while standing on a Bosu ball with your feet hip-width apart. With your knees in line with your toes and your core working, lower yourself into a squat. Take a few moments to hold this posture, then stand back up.

Including Core Strength in Everyday Tasks

- **Standing Core Engagement:** Even when you're not exercising, work on using your core muscles throughout the day. Whether you're doing the dishes at home or in line at the grocery store, pay attention to your posture and bring your belly button in toward your spine.
- **Functional Movements:** Seek ways to include exercises that strengthen your core into your regular routine. For instance, consider squatting down and using your core muscles to raise the

object instead than bending over to pick it up.

Examples of Routines and Exercises

- Complete Body Isometric Exercise: Do each exercise for 30–60 seconds, pausing for 15–30 seconds in between. Do the circuit two or three times again.

Every side of the plank is a plank.

Bird Dog Hold: Superman Holds (either side)

Daily Upkeep of the Core Routine: Complete each exercise for 10–20 seconds without stopping. Do the circuit two or three times again.

Prominent Core Participation

- Balance on Just One Leg (each leg)
- Bosu Ball Squat Hold Functional Motions (such as bending down to pick something up).

In summary

Your balance, stability, and general functional strength will all improve if you incorporate isometric core exercises into your full-body workouts and everyday activities. Throughout each exercise, keep in mind to maintain good form, contract your core muscles, and pay attention to your body's cues. Your core strength and general level of fitness will increase with time if you are consistent and dedicated. Continue your fantastic effort!

Chapter 7

Progression and Modification

We'll look at how to advance and adapt your isometric core workouts in this chapter so you can keep pushing your muscles and improving your overall fitness level. There are techniques you may employ to keep your workouts interesting and productive, regardless of your level of experience. Let's get started and investigate how to advance your training.

Increasing Intensity Gradually

You will continue to experience improvements if you gradually raise the intensity of your workouts as you get stronger and more accustomed to your isometric exercises. There are various ways to accomplish this, including:

Extending the time for every exercise:

To begin, hold each exercise for a few more seconds than you did in earlier training sessions. Increase the time gradually as you get more comfortable until you can hold each exercise for at least 60 seconds.

Increasing the resistance:

Use weights, resistance bands, or other props to make your workouts more challenging. To add resistance to your core muscles during a plank or side plank, for instance, you can grasp a dumbbell or kettle bell.

Attempting more difficult variations:

Try even more difficult iterations of your best workouts to challenge yourself and target various muscle areas. To further engage your core muscles, try a side plank with a leg lift or a single-arm plank.

Adapting Exercises to Various Degrees of Fitness

It's critical to keep in mind that not everyone is at the same level of fitness, and that what suits one individual may not suit another. It's crucial to adjust your workouts to fit your unique demands and capabilities because of this. The following advice can be used to change exercises:

- **Lower the intensity:** Don't be scared to lower the intensity if an activity seems too difficult. For instance, you can hold a wall sit for a shorter period of time or do a plank on your knees rather than your toes.
- **Put form first:** Pay attention to maintaining appropriate form and technique during an activity rather than trying to force through a difficult workout. In the long run, this will help you stay injury-free and maximize your efforts.

Above all, pay attention to what your body is telling you and respect its limitations. As soon as something hurts or doesn't feel right, stop using it and get medical advice.

Examples of Routines and Exercises

Simple Isometric Exercise: Three sets of 20-second holds for the plank

Each side of the plank: three sets of 15-second holds

Hold Superman: three sets of twenty seconds

Hold the bird dog three times for fifteen seconds on each side.

Advanced Isometric Exercise: Three sets of 30-second holds for each side of the single-arm plank

- Three sets of 20-second holds for each side of the side plank with leg lift.
- Three sets of 25-second holds for the weighted Superman hold
- Holding the Bosu Ball Squat with a Resistance Band: three sets of thirty seconds

In summary

You'll keep improving your fitness and accomplishing your goals if you progressively up the intensity of your workouts and alter the routines to fit your unique needs. Always pay attention to correct form, pay attention to your body, and enjoy yourself while working out. You won't believe what you can do if you put in the effort and are consistent!

Chapter8

Staying Motivated and Consistent

This chapter will cover techniques for maintaining your isometric core training regimen's consistency and motivation. Developing a regular exercise routine is essential to reaching your fitness objectives and sustaining long-term success. Let's get started and learn how to maintain motivation while pursuing your fitness goals.

Establish Specific, Achievable Goals

Establishing attainable objectives for oneself is one of the best strategies to maintain motivation. A well-defined goal to strive for, such as enhancing your endurance, hitting a particular milestone, or strengthening your core, will help you stay motivated and focused. Make careful to divide your objectives into more manageable chunks and acknowledge your accomplishments as you go.

Find Things to Do That You Enjoy

It should be enjoyable and something you look forward to doing to exercise instead of feeling like a duty. Maintaining motivation and consistency during your workouts will be difficult if you're not enjoying yourself. Try out a variety of isometric workouts and activities until you discover one that you really enjoy. There's something for everyone out there, be it a lone outdoor trip, a virtual workout, or a group fitness class.

Stir Things Up

Variety is essential to maintaining motivation for your workouts and the flavor of life. Make changes to your regimen to keep your workouts interesting and fresh rather than following the same one every day. Experiment with various isometric exercise forms, rearrange the sequence in which you perform your exercises, and discover novel training settings. This will keep you from getting bored as well as pushing your body in novel ways as you continue to move closer to your objectives.

Locate a Partner for Accountability

It can be help to have someone hold you accountable if you want to maintain your motivation and consistency during your workouts. Having someone to check in with and discuss your progress with, be it a friend, family member, or personal trainer, can help you stay accountable and on track towards your goals. Plus, working out with a friend is much more enjoyable!

Take Care of Yourself

Maintaining motivation and consistency in your workouts requires taking care of your body and mind. As part of your total exercise regimen, remember to give rest, recuperation, and relaxation first priority. This include obtaining adequate rest, feeding your body wholesome foods, and setting aside time for relaxation and stress relief. Recall that taking care of oneself is essential to leading a balanced and healthy lifestyle, not selfishness.

Honor Your Achievements

Lastly, remember to recognize and honor your accomplishments along the route. Take the time to recognize and celebrate your accomplishments, whether they are hitting a new personal record, perfecting a difficult activity, or maintaining your fitness schedule for a predetermined amount of time. Acknowledging your efforts and accomplishments will keep you inspired and driven to keep working toward your objectives.

Maintaining a healthy and active lifestyle and attaining long-term success with your isometric core training regimen depend on your ability to stay motivated and consistent. You'll be well on your way to achieving your fitness objectives and leading the best possible life by creating clear goals, engaging in enjoyable activities, varying up your workouts, finding an accountability partner, taking care of yourself, and celebrating your accomplishments.

Chapter 9

Nutritional Tips for Supporting Core Health

Greetings from Chapter 9! We'll look at the role diet plays in maintaining core health and giving your body the energy it needs to function at its peak in this chapter. You may maximize the benefits of your isometric workout regimen by maintaining a strong and healthy core through the consumption of a well-balanced, nutrient-rich diet. Now let's get started and learn some dietary advice for maintaining fundamental health.

Providing Energy for Your Exercises

Your body requires fuel to function at its peak during workouts, much like an automobile needs fuel to run. Your muscles will have more energy to perform your isometric exercises if you have a balanced meal or snack before your workout. About 30 to 60 minutes prior to your activity, try to have a balance of carbohydrates and protein, like a Greek yogurt with berries or a banana with almond butter.

Drinking Water

Maintaining optimal performance and promoting general health, particularly core health, require drinking enough of water. When it comes to maintaining body temperature, lubricating joints, and delivering nutrients to cells, water is essential. To stay adequately hydrated, make sure you drink lots of water throughout the day, especially before, during, and after your workouts.

Put Whole Foods First

Focus on packing your plate with full, nutrient-dense foods that feed your body from the inside out to support core wellness. A wide range of vital nutrients can be obtained by selecting a variety of fruits, vegetables, lean proteins, whole grains, and healthy fats. Not only can colorful fruits and vegetables offer taste and diversity to your meals, but they also include essential vitamins, minerals, and antioxidants that promote general health and wellbeing.

Consume A Lot of Protein

Building and mending muscles, especially the muscles in your core, require protein. To promote muscle growth and repair, incorporate a source of protein into each of your meals and snacks. Lean meats, chicken, fish, eggs, dairy products, tofu, tempeh, beans, lentils, and legumes are all excellent sources of protein.

Remind Yourself of Fiber

Another essential ingredient for maintaining general digestive health and function is fiber. Consume a diet high in fruits, vegetables, whole grains, nuts, seeds, and legumes, as well as other fiber-rich foods. Fiber promotes a healthy weight, keeps your digestive tract functioning normally, and helps you avoid constipation—all of which are critical for keeping your core strong and healthy.

Limit Processed Foods and Added Sugars

Your attempts to keep a strong and healthy core can be undermined by processed foods and added sugars, which can have a disastrous effect on your health. These meals can lead to weight gain, inflammation, and digestive problems since they are frequently heavy in calories, bad fats, and refined carbohydrates. Rather, prioritize eating as many whole, minimally processed foods as you can, and cut less on sugary snacks, sodas, and processed snacks.

In order to maintain core health and provide your body the energy it needs to function at its peak during isometric activities, nutrition is essential. You may sustain your general health and well-being for years to come by eating a balanced diet, drinking plenty of water, and emphasizing whole, nutrient-dense foods.

Conclusion

Congratulations for finishing this exploration of seniors' isometric core workouts! We have covered the principles of isometric exercises, the structure of the core muscles, critical safety issues, and useful advice for incorporating these exercises into your everyday practice throughout this book.

You now have a thorough grasp of the advantages isometric exercises can provide seniors in terms of increased stability, strength, and general wellbeing. You now know how to target different muscle groups in the core with a range of exercises, and you also know how to advance and adjust your workouts to fit your unique requirements and capabilities.

Recall that the secret to enjoying the fruits of your labor is constancy. Maintain your motivation, your consistency, and—above all—pay attention to your body. No matter how tiny, acknowledge your accomplishments along the road, and don't be embarrassed to seek advice or assistance when you need it.

Remember that enjoying the journey is just as important as reaching your destination when you continue on your fitness path. Above all, enjoy yourself while working out, embrace the process, and maintain your curiosity. Your body is capable of incredible things, and you can live your best life and reach your fitness goals if you put in the necessary effort and persistence.

I appreciate you coming along on this journey with me as we explore the realm of senior isometric core workouts. With each plank, side twist, and deep breath, I hope you are motivated and equipped to take control of your health and well-being. To a more robust, well-being, and joyous version of yourself!

Continue to move, to smile, and to shine brightly.